Epsom Salt

Holistic Epsom Salt Recipes & Uses for Health, Beauty, Relaxation, Home & Garden

By Cassia Albinson

Copyright © Cassia Albinson 2016

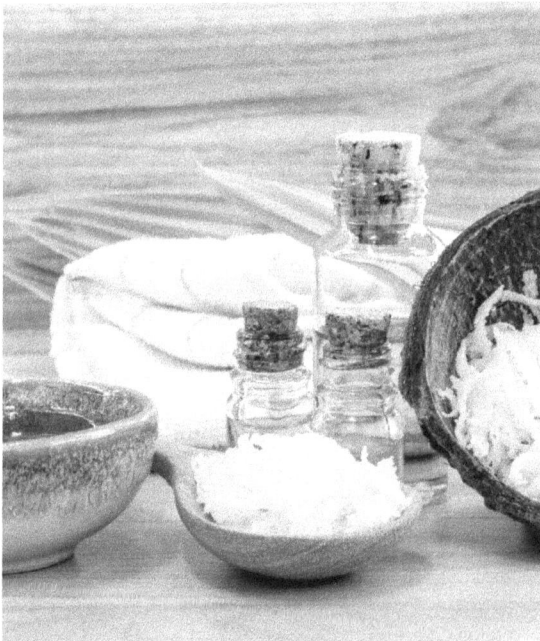

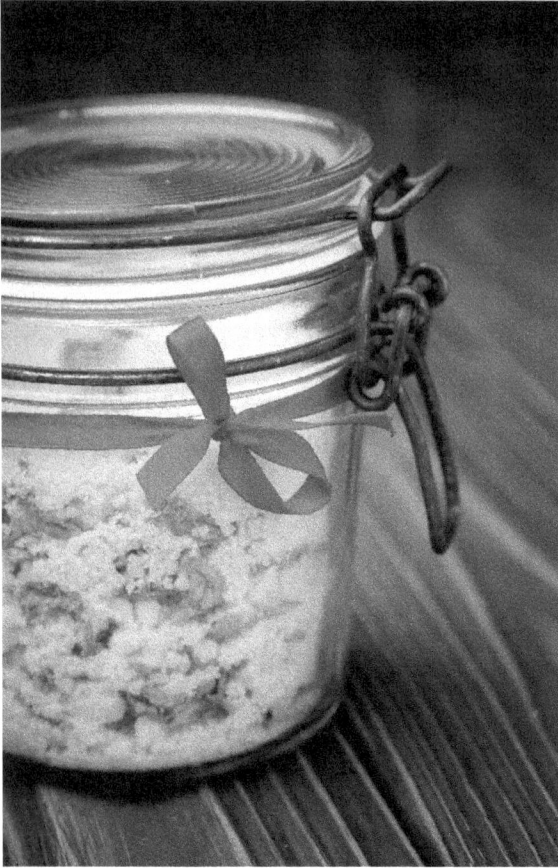

Epsom Salt- Holistic Epsom Salt Recipes & Uses

Contents

Introduction

When you hear the word "salt" you probably picture a salt shaker filled with tiny white grains – the kind of salt you use to season your favorite meals. While this may be the most commonly used salt, there are actually many kinds of salt. Not only do different types of salt have different flavors and colors, but they have different purposes as well. One type of salt that you may or may not be familiar with is called Epsom salt. Epsom salt is not typically used for cooking but it does have a wide variety of benefits and applications in the fields of health, beauty, gardening, crafts, and more.

In this book you will receive an in-depth introduction to Epsom salt and its many benefits. You will learn where it comes from and what it is exactly. You will also receive an overview of the health, medical, home, and beauty applications for this wonderful salt. Finally, you will receive a collection of quick and easy recipes using Epsom salt that you can try for yourself. So, if you are ready to learn more about Epsom salt, just turn the page and keep reading!

What is Epsom Salt?

The first thing you need to know about Epsom salt is that it is actually called "magnesium sulfate". Magnesium sulfate is a type of inorganic salt, a chemical compound, that contains magnesium as well as sulfur and oxygen – the chemical formula for this compound is $MgSO_4$. You can probably see why it is more commonly referred to as Epsom salt! The name for this compound comes from a saline spring located in an area of Surrey, England known as Epsom which contains high levels of the pure mineral compound. Epsom salt has a great many benefits and applications and it has been used for hundreds of years by many different cultures.

Benefits of Epsom Salt

The benefits of Epsom salt are vast and varied. Because Epsom salt is actually a mineral compound and not technically a salt, it is generally not used for culinary purposes. It can, however, provide many beneficial properties that can soothe the mind and body as well as the soul. Epsom salt has the ability to relax the human nervous system, to soothe aches and pains, to speed healing, and to draw toxins out of the body. This mineral compound also has stress-relieving properties. <u>To give you a better idea what Epsom salt can really do, here is a list of its benefits</u>:

- Replenishes magnesium levels in the body which can help boost mood and provide a calming, relaxing benefit.
- Encourages ATP production which increases both energy and stamina.
- Reduces the effects of adrenaline to help with relaxation and to reduce irritability.
- May help to improve sleep and concentration.
- Eases pain and reduced inflammation for the treatment of sore muscles, aches, or pains.
- May help to heal cuts and other minor injuries more quickly.
- Soaking may help to soften skin and neutralize foot odor.
- May help to regulate electrolyte levels, boosting the function of nerves, enzymes, and muscles in the body.
- Helps the body to utilize calcium more efficiently and serves as a conductor for electrical impulses in the body.
- May help to improve heart health and to prevent stroke and heart disease by boosting blood circulation, improving elasticity of the arteries, and preventing blood clots.
- Helps balance magnesium and sulfate levels in the body which may improve insulin response and utilization, reduced risk for diabetes.

- May help to detoxify the colon and provide relief from constipation when taking internally.
- Could help to flush heavy metals and other toxins from the body through the skin using the process of reverse osmosis.

Now that you know a little bit more about the general benefits for Epsom salt you may be curious to know exactly how it works. Dissolving Epsom salt in water for a soak or a bath is the most common way to use this compound but there are other options as well. In the next few sections you will learn about specific uses for Epsom salt and you will receive some quick and easy recipes as well.

Health and Medical Uses for Epsom Salt

Magnesium sulfate, or Epsom salt, can be used both internally and externally for health and medicinal benefits. External uses for this compound generally involve dissolving the compound in water and then soaking in it – magnesium and sulfate can both be absorbed through the skin. Some of the health and medicinal uses for Epsom salt include the following:

- Soaking to relieve the symptoms of athlete's foot – may also reduce foot odor.
- Bathing to treat toenail fungus or other fungal foot problems.
- Made into a compress to relieve pain and discomfort for sore muscles.
- Soaking or made into a paste to help draw out a splinter.
- Bathing or soaking to reduce pain and swelling for sprains and bruises.
- Soaking to reduce inflammation caused by gout.
- Providing itch relief for poison ivy and/or sunburn.
- Bathing can help to soothe abdominal cramps and alleviate headaches.
- Helps to regulate fluid retention in the cells, balancing electrolytes.

- Soaking may improve circulation to help reduce blood clots and lower blood pressure to improve cardiovascular health.
- Improves the body's ability to produce and utilize insulin efficiently.

Home and Beauty Uses for Epsom Salt

Not only does Epsom salt provide a great many benefits for general health and wellness, but it can also be used for a variety of home and beauty applications. Epsom salt can be made into homemade scrubs to exfoliate the skin or even in homemade cleaners for your face and body. <u>Some of the top home and beauty uses for Epsom salt include the following</u>:

- Rubbing salts over damp skin can help to remove dead skin cells, making skin softer and healthier.
- Can be used as an exfoliating face mask or scrub to remove oil from pores and to remove blackheads.
- May help to add volume to hair or may help to remove product buildup.
- Can be mixed with baby oil to create a homemade moisturizing hand cleanser.
- May be used in a soak to facilitation relaxation and stress relief.
- Can be made into homemade bath salts for aromatherapy and relaxation.
- May help plants grow larger and greener, facilitates natural growth.
- Can be used as a natural fertilizer to help plants grow larger and produce more flowers.

- May help to prevent slugs and other insect pests from entering the house.
- Can be used as a homemade scrub for bathroom tile and grout.
- May be combined with other ingredients to create a natural pesticide/insecticide.
- Can help to remove detergent buildup from the washing machine tub.

Spa and Beauty Epsom Salt Recipes

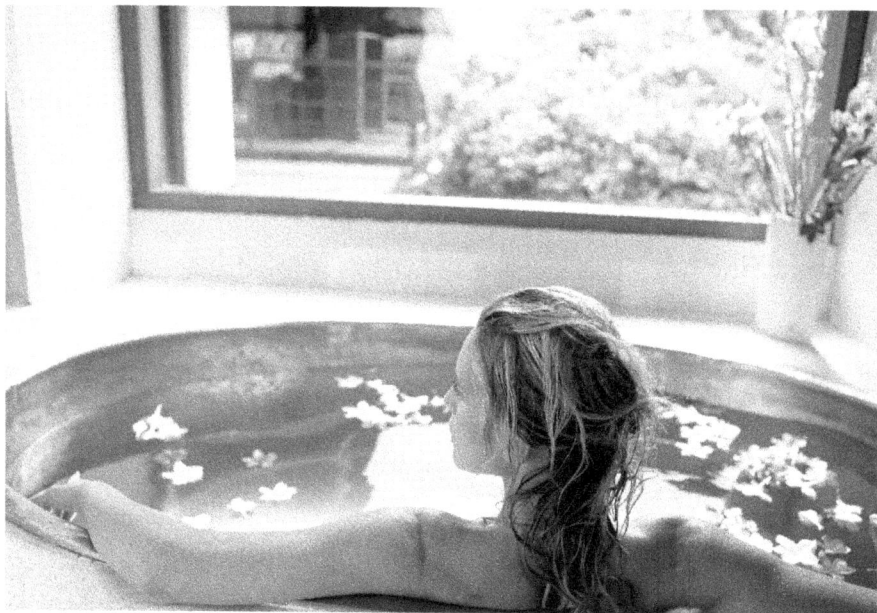

Relaxing Bath Salt Blend

There is no better way to settle down at the end of the day than with a relaxing bath. This relaxing bath salt blend will have your worries and fears swirling away down the drain.

Ingredients:

- 8 ounces Epsom salt
- 10 drops lavender essential oil
- 3 drops chamomile essential oil

Instructions:

1. Combine the Epsom salt and essential oils in a non-reactive bowl.
2. Mix the ingredients well until thoroughly combined.
3. Pour the bath salts into a glass jar and cover tightly with the lid.
4. Store in a cool, dark place until ready to use.
5. To use, add a handful of bath salts to a running bath and stir by hand until the salts are dissolved.
6. Soak for at least 30 minutes then towel dry.

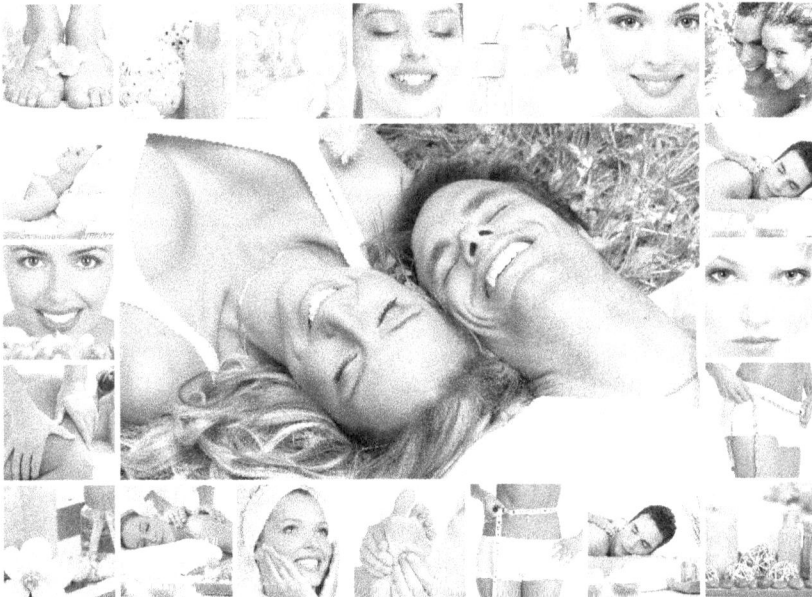

Aromatherapy Pedicure Soak

This aromatherapy pedicure soak is soothing and relaxing, plus it will help to soften your skin. After soaking, rub your feet with an Epsom salt scrub to maximize the benefits.

Ingredients:

- 2 quarts warm water
- ½ cup Epsom salt
- 3 drops eucalyptus essential oil
- 3 drops tea tree essential oil

Instructions:

1. Pour two quarts of warm water into a basin then stir in the Epsom salt.
2. Add the essential oils and swirl well to distribute.
3. Place the basin on the floor and soak your feet for 15 to 20 minutes.
4. Remove your feet from the basin and scrub your feet well with an Epsom salt scrub.
5. Rinse your feet well with warm water then towel dry.

Floral Coconut Oil Salt Scrub

This floral coconut oil salt scrub is made with just a few simple ingredients but it will leave your skin feeling fresh and clean. Use it daily for the best results!

Ingredients:

- 2 cups cold-pressed coconut oil
- 1 cup Epsom salt
- 10 drops jasmine essential oil
- 10 drops lavender essential oil

Instructions:

1. Combine the coconut oil, Epsom salt and essential oils in a mixing bowl.
2. Stir the ingredients until thoroughly combined.
3. Spoon the mixture into a glass jar and cover tightly with the lid.
4. When ready to use, dampen your skin then apply a small amount of the scrub.
5. Gently rub the scrub into your skin in a circular motion then rinse and pat dry.

Vanilla Hair Volumizer

If you want lovely, luscious locks of hair then you should try this natural hair volumizer. Using your favorite conditioner and some Epsom salt you can make a natural product that will give your hair the volume you crave.

Ingredients:

- 2 tablespoons conditioner
- 2 tablespoons Epsom salt
- ½ teaspoon vanilla extract

Instructions:

1. Warm the conditioner in the microwave in a small bowl.
2. Stir in the Epsom salt and the vanilla extract.
3. Dampen your hair in the shower then work in the volumizer.
4. Let the volumizer soak in for 20 minutes then rinse and towel dry.

Simple Bath Bomb

If you want to experience luxury without paying the luxury price tag, these simple bath bombs are worth a try! Just add your choice of essential oils or herbs for a nice scent.

Ingredients:

- 1 cup baking soda
- ½ cup Epsom salt
- ½ cup citric acid
- ½ tablespoon olive oil
- ½ tablespoon water
- 1 teaspoon vanilla extract

Instructions:

1. Stir together the baking soda, Epsom salt, and citric acid in a mixing bowl.
2. In a separate bowl, whisk together the olive oil, water, and vanilla extract.
3. Stir the liquid ingredients into the dry ingredients and mix well by hand until thoroughly combined.
4. Add more water, if needed, to make the mixture stick together.
5. Divide the mixture among small silicone molds, pressing it firmly.
6. Let the mold sit for 24 to 48 hours until completely hardened.

7. Remove the bath bombs from the mold and store in an airtight container for up to 2 weeks.

8. To use, add one bath bomb to a hot bath and let it fizz!

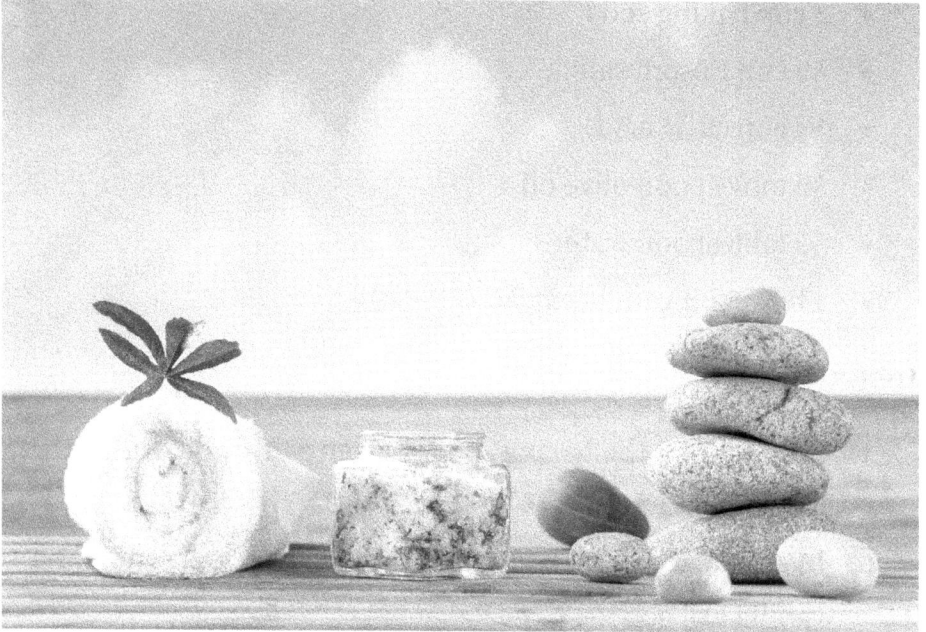

Epsom Salt Face Mask

If your skin is oily or covered with blemishes, this all-natural Epsom salt face mask may be just what you need. Apply this mask daily for the best results.

Ingredients:

- ¼ cup powdered milk
- ¼ cup fresh lemon juice
- 1 tablespoon cognac
- ½ teaspoon Epsom salt
- 1 egg, whisked well

Instructions:

1. Combine all of the ingredients in a small bowl.
2. Whisk everything together until smooth and well combined.
3. Dampen the skin on your face then apply the mask in a thin layer.
4. Let the mask soak for 15 minutes or so then rinse and pat dry.

Soothing Bath Salt Blend

This soothing bath salt blend is just what you need to relieve your muscle aches and pains. Simply stir the salts into a hot bath then soak for 30 minutes.

Ingredients:

- 8 ounces Epsom salt
- 10 drops lavender essential oil
- 3 drops eucalyptus essential oil

Instructions:

1. Combine the Epsom salt and essential oils in a non-reactive bowl.
2. Mix the ingredients well until thoroughly combined.
3. Pour the bath salts into a glass jar and cover tightly with the lid.
4. Store in a cool, dark place until ready to use.
5. To use, add a handful of bath salts to a running bath and stir by hand until the salts are dissolved.
6. Soak for at least 30 minutes then towel dry.

Sleep-Promoting Pedicure Soak

After a long day, this sleep-promoting pedicure soak will help you to wind down and get ready to sleep. Plus, your feet will be clean and soft as an added bonus!

Ingredients:

- 2 quarts warm water
- ½ cup Epsom salt
- 3 drops rose essential oil
- 3 drops geranium essential oil
- 3 drops lavender essential oil

Instructions:

1. Pour two quarts of warm water into a basin then stir in the Epsom salt.
2. Add the essential oils and swirl well to distribute.
3. Place the basin on the floor and soak your feet for 15 to 20 minutes.
4. Remove your feet from the basin and scrub your feet well with an Epsom salt scrub.
5. Rinse your feet well with warm water then towel dry.

Easy Hairspray Remover

After a night on the town your hair is probably full of hairspray or other hair products. Rather than subjecting your hair to hot water to get rid of it, try this easy hairspray remover made with water, lemon juice and Epsom salt.

Ingredients:

- 2 quarts water
- ½ cup fresh lemon juice
- ½ cup Epsom salt

Instructions:

1. Combine the water, lemon juice and Epsom salt in a large bowl.
2. Stir well then let the mixture sit overnight, covered.
3. The next day, pour the mixture into your hair and work it in.
4. Soak for 20 minutes then shampoo and rinse as normal.

Invigorating Salt Facial Scrub

This invigorating salt scrub will not only leave your skin looking fresh and youthful, but it will give you a boost of energy as well!

Ingredients:

- 1 cup Epsom salt
- ½ cup jojoba oil
- 10 drops grapefruit essential oil
- 4 drops bergamot essential oil
- 2 drops lemon essential oil

Instructions:

1. Combine the Epsom salt and essential oils in a non-reactive bowl.
2. Mix the ingredients well until thoroughly combined.
3. Pour the scrub into a glass jar and cover tightly with the lid.

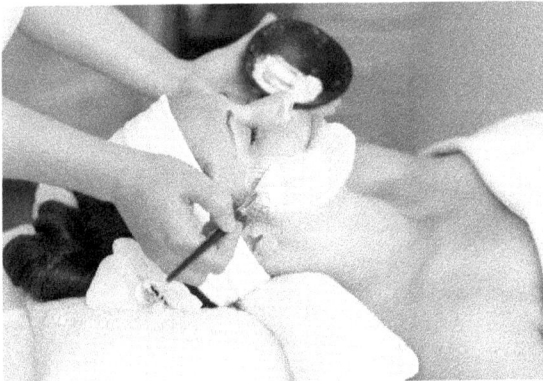

Clarifying Hair Volumizer

This clarifying hair volumizer does more than just add volume to your hair – the essential oil blend will also help to clear your mind of distractions so you can focus.

Ingredients:

- 2 tablespoons conditioner
- 2 tablespoons Epsom salt
- 3 drops thyme essential oil
- 3 drops rosemary essential oil
- 3 drops peppermint essential oil

Instructions:

1. Warm the conditioner in the microwave in a small bowl.
2. Stir in the Epsom salt and the essential oils.
3. Dampen your hair in the shower then work in the volumizer.
4. Let the volumizer soak in for 20 minutes then rinse and towel dry.

Balancing Bath Bombs

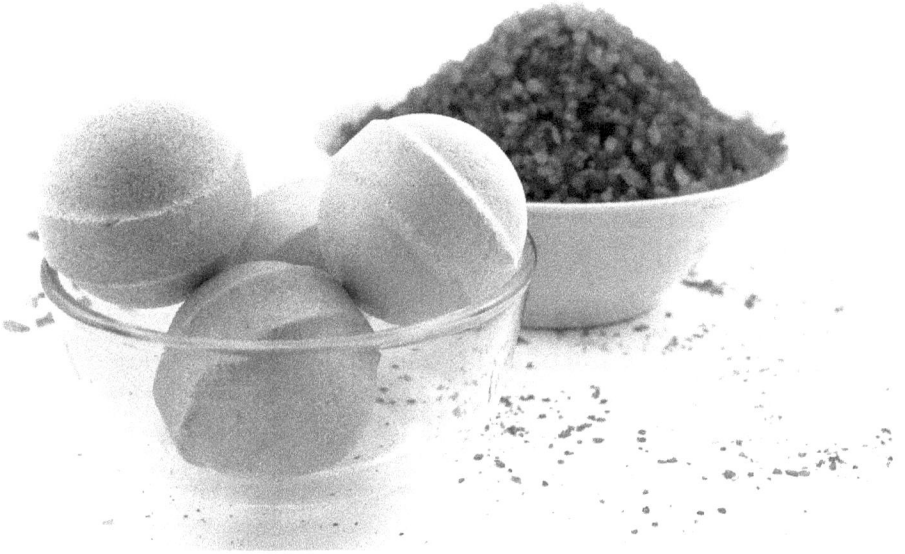

Scented with a combination of sage, mint, and tea tree oil, these bath bombs release a calming and balancing aroma while you soak in the hot bath.

Ingredients:

- 1 cup baking soda
- ½ cup Epsom salt
- ½ cup citric acid
- ½ tablespoon olive oil
- ½ tablespoon water
- 1 teaspoon vanilla extract
- 10 drops sage essential oil
- 5 drops mint essential oil

- 5 drops tea tree essential oil

Instructions:

1. Stir together the baking soda, Epsom salt, and citric acid in a mixing bowl.
2. In a separate bowl, whisk together the olive oil, water, and vanilla extract.
3. Stir the liquid ingredients into the dry ingredients and mix well by hand until thoroughly combined.
4. Add the essential oils and add more water, if needed, to make the mixture stick together.
5. Divide the mixture among small silicone molds, pressing it firmly.
6. Let the mold sit for 24 to 48 hours until completely hardened.
7. Remove the bath bombs from the mold and store in an airtight container for up to 2 weeks.
8. To use, add one bath bomb to a hot bath and let it fizz!

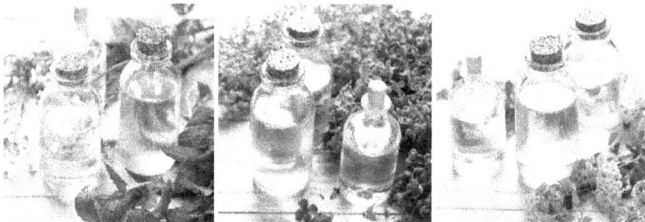

Epsom Salt Mask for Dry Skin

If your skin is dry it could be a sign of dehydration. Not only should you drink more water but you should try this Epsom salt mask to rehydrate your skin and to restore your youthful glow.

Ingredients:

- ¼ cup finely grated carrot
- 1 ½ teaspoons mayonnaise
- ½ teaspoon Epsom salt
- ½ teaspoon honey

Instructions:

1. Combine all of the ingredients in a small bowl.
2. Whisk everything together until smooth and well combined.
3. Dampen the skin on your face then apply the mask in a thin layer.
4. Let the mask soak for 15 minutes or so then rinse and pat dry.

Energizing Bath Salt Blend

It may seem strange to take a bath as a way to boost your energy but this bath salt blend made with rosemary and peppermint essential oils are sure to put a little pep in your step.

Ingredients:

- 8 ounces Epsom salt
- 10 drops rosemary essential oil
- 4 drops peppermint essential oil

Instructions:

1. Combine the Epsom salt and essential oils in a non-reactive bowl.
2. Mix the ingredients well until thoroughly combined.
3. Pour the bath salts into a glass jar and cover tightly with the lid.
4. Store in a cool, dark place until ready to use.
5. To use, add a handful of bath salts to a running bath and stir by hand until the salts are dissolved.
6. Soak for at least 30 minutes then towel dry.

Holiday-Scented Pedicure Soak

This scented pedicure soak is sure to get you into the holiday spirit, plus it will leave your feet feeling soft and renewed. So what are you waiting for, give it a try!

Ingredients:

- 2 quarts warm water
- ½ cup Epsom salt
- 2 drops cinnamon essential oil
- 2 drops patchouli essential oil
- 2 drops orange essential oil
- 2 drops clove essential oil

Instructions:

1. Pour two quarts of warm water into a basin then stir in the Epsom salt.
2. Add the essential oils and swirl well to distribute.
3. Place the basin on the floor and soak your feet for 15 to 20 minutes.
4. Remove your feet from the basin and scrub your feet well with an Epsom salt scrub.
5. Rinse your feet well with warm water then towel dry.

Lemon Rosemary Exfoliating Scrub

If you are looking for an all-natural beauty routine that will leave your skin smooth and supply, give this lemon rosemary salt scrub a try.

Ingredients:

- 10 tablespoons Epsom salt
- 2 tablespoons olive oil
- ¼ cup fresh lemon juice
- 1 tablespoon dried rosemary

Instructions:

1. Combine the olive oil, Epsom salt and lemon juice in a mixing bowl.
2. Stir the ingredients until thoroughly combined then add the rosemary.
3. Spoon the mixture into a glass jar and cover tightly with the lid.
4. When ready to use, dampen your skin then apply a small amount of the scrub.
5. Gently rub the scrub into your skin in a circular motion then rinse and pat dry.

Mood-Lifting Hair Volumizer

When you've had a tough day it might make you feel better to pamper yourself a bit with this homemade hair volumizer. As an added bonus, it is made with essential oils that will help to naturally lift your mood.

Ingredients:

- 2 tablespoons conditioner
- 2 tablespoons Epsom salt
- 3 drops bergamot essential oil
- 3 drops lavender essential oil
- 3 drops geranium essential oil

Instructions:

1. Warm the conditioner in the microwave in a small bowl.
2. Stir in the Epsom salt and the essential oils.
3. Dampen your hair in the shower then work in the volumizer.
4. Let the volumizer soak in for 20 minutes then rinse and towel dry.

Uplifting Bath Bombs

If you are feeling stressed and rundown, these uplifting bath bombs may be just what you need. Toss one into a hot bath them climb in and relax.

Ingredients:

- 1 cup baking soda
- ½ cup Epsom salt
- ½ cup citric acid
- ½ tablespoon olive oil
- ½ tablespoon water
- 1 teaspoon vanilla extract
- 5 drops orange essential oil
- 5 drops clove essential oil
- 5 drops lemon essential oil
- 5 drops cedarwood essential oil

Instructions:

1. Stir together the baking soda, Epsom salt, and citric acid in a mixing bowl.
2. In a separate bowl, whisk together the olive oil, water, and vanilla extract.
3. Stir the liquid ingredients into the dry ingredients and mix well by hand until thoroughly combined.
4. Add the essential oils and add more water, if needed, to make the mixture stick together.

5. Divide the mixture among small silicone molds, pressing it firmly.
6. Let the mold sit for 24 to 48 hours until completely hardened.
7. Remove the bath bombs from the mold and store in an airtight container for up to 2 weeks.
8. To use, add one bath bomb to a hot bath and let it fizz!

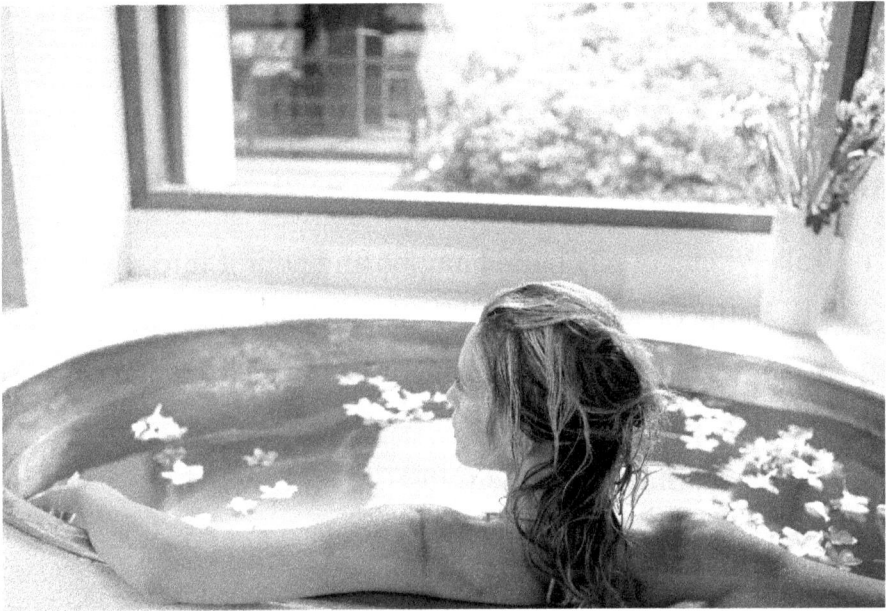

Hair Oil Remover

If you have naturally oily hair you may feel as though you've tried everything to fix it. This easy hair oil remover is not expensive and it isn't made with fancy ingredients but it will definitely get the job done. Just try it for yourself!

Ingredients:

- ½ cup oily hair shampoo
- ½ cup Epsom salt
- Apple cider vinegar, as needed

Instructions:

1. Take ½ cup of oily hair shampoo and pour it into a bowl.
2. Stir in the Epsom salt until thoroughly combined.
3. With dry hair, apply 1 tablespoon of the mixture and work it through.
4. Rinse your hair with cold water.
5. Pour the apple cider vinegar over your hair and let it soak for 10 minutes.
6. Rinse your hair well with cold water then towel dry.

Stress-Relieving Bath Salt Blend

If the stress of your busy life is starting to get you down, take a moment for yourself and enjoy a hot, relaxing bath with this stress-relieving bath salt blend.

Ingredients:

- 8 ounces Epsom salt
- 10 drops rose essential oil
- 3 drops bergamot essential oil

Instructions:

1. Combine the Epsom salt and essential oils in a non-reactive bowl.
2. Mix the ingredients well until thoroughly combined.
3. Pour the bath salts into a glass jar and cover tightly with the lid.
4. Store in a cool, dark place until ready to use.
5. To use, add a handful of bath salts to a running bath and stir by hand until the salts are dissolved.
6. Soak for at least 30 minutes then towel dry.

Energizing Pedicure Soak

If you are starting to feel tired and run down, give yourself 15 to 20 minutes to soak your feet with this energizing pedicure soak. Not only will your feet be soft and exfoliated after but you will have renewed energy levels as well!

Ingredients:

- 2 quarts warm water
- ½ cup Epsom salt
- 4 drops peppermint essential oil
- 4 drops wild orange essential oil

Instructions:

1. Pour two quarts of warm water into a basin then stir in the Epsom salt.
2. Add the essential oils and swirl well to distribute.
3. Place the basin on the floor and soak your feet for 15 to 20 minutes.
4. Remove your feet from the basin and scrub your feet well with an Epsom salt scrub.
5. Rinse your feet well with warm water then towel dry.

Lovely Lavender Scrub

This lovely lavender scrub takes just a few minutes to put together and you will have enough of it to last several weeks. Enjoy the soothing scent of lavender as you wash your face.

Ingredients:

- 2 cups cold-pressed coconut oil
- 1 cup Epsom salt
- 10 drops lavender essential oil
- 5 drops rose essential oil
- 5 drops geranium essential oil

Instructions:

1. Combine the coconut oil, Epsom salt and essential oils in a mixing bowl.
2. Stir the ingredients until thoroughly combined.
3. Spoon the mixture into a glass jar and cover tightly with the lid.
4. When ready to use, dampen your skin then apply a small amount of the scrub.
5. Gently rub the scrub into your skin in a circular motion then rinse and pat dry.

Sweet and Sensual Hair Volumizer

There is no better way to pamper yourself than with this natural hair volumizer. This recipe is made with essential oils that will help you to get into the mood as well.

Ingredients:

- 2 tablespoons conditioner
- 2 tablespoons Epsom salt
- 5 drops sandalwood essential oil
- 2 drops vanilla essential oil
- 1 drop jasmine essential oil

Instructions:

1. Warm the conditioner in the microwave in a small bowl.
2. Stir in the Epsom salt and the essential oils.
3. Dampen your hair in the shower then work in the volumizer.
4. Let the volumizer soak in for 20 minutes then rinse and towel dry.

Mind-Clearing Bath Bombs

It is easy to become overwhelmed with stress during our daily lives but these mind-clearing bath bombs will help you push through the fog.

Ingredients:

- 1 cup baking soda
- ½ cup Epsom salt
- ½ cup citric acid
- ½ tablespoon olive oil
- ½ tablespoon water
- 1 teaspoon vanilla extract
- 12 drops rosemary essential oil
- 12 drops lemon essential oil

Instructions:

1. Stir together the baking soda, Epsom salt, and citric acid in a mixing bowl.
2. In a separate bowl, whisk together the olive oil, water, and vanilla extract.
3. Stir the liquid ingredients into the dry ingredients and mix well by hand until thoroughly combined.
4. Add the essential oils and add more water, if needed, to make the mixture stick together.
5. Divide the mixture among small silicone molds, pressing it firmly.

6. Let the mold sit for 24 to 48 hours until completely hardened.
7. Remove the bath bombs from the mold and store in an airtight container for up to 2 weeks.
8. To use, add one bath bomb to a hot bath and let it fizz!

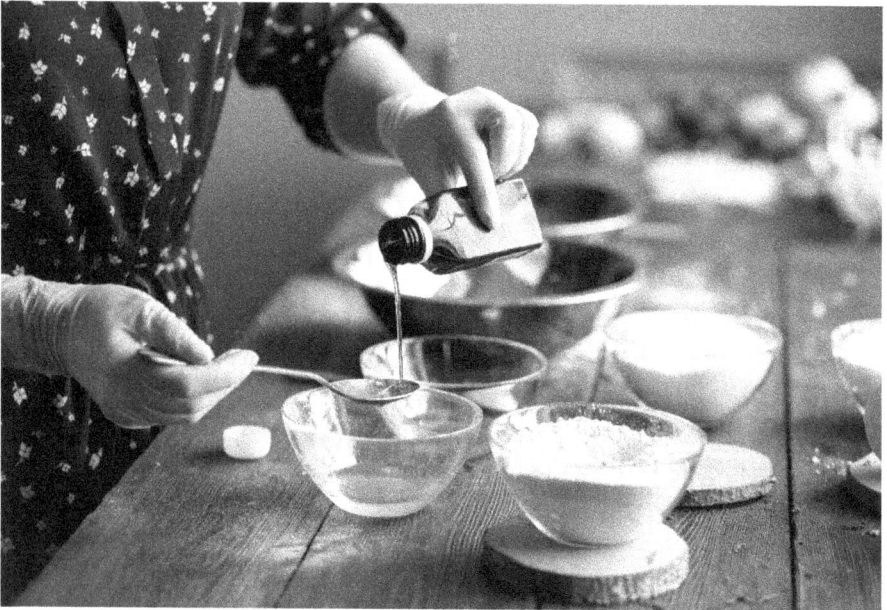

Health and Medical Epsom Salt Recipes

Splinter Removal Paste

Removing splinters can be difficult, especially if they are very small or very deep. With this splinter removal paste you can save yourself the pain and frustration of digging around.

Ingredients:

- 8 ounces hot water
- 1 teaspoon Epsom salt

Instructions:

1. Pour the water into a small bowl and stir in the Epsom salt.
2. Stir the mixture until the salt is completely dissolved.
3. Transfer the solution to the refrigerator and chill for 20 minutes.
4. Clean the affected area and pat dry then apply a layer of paste.
5. Cover the paste with a bandage and check after 30 minutes.

Poison Ivy Relief Compress

Some people do not have a reaction to poison ivy but others are not so lucky. If you are one of the unlucky ones you'll be glad to have this recipe on hand – it is simple to prepare and it can help to relieve the pain and itching of poison ivy.

Ingredients:

- 1 cup cold water
- 2 tablespoons Epsom salt
- 1 drop tea tree essential oil
- 1 drop lavender essential oil

Instructions:

1. Combine the cold water and Epsom salt in a small bowl.
2. Stir until the salt is dissolved then stir in the essential oil.
3. Soak a washcloth in the solution then lay it over the affected area.
4. Let the washcloth sit on the area until it is no longer cold.
5. Repeat this treatment as needed.

Post-Natal Bath Bombs

After giving birth the only thing you want to do is rest and relax. With these post-natal bath bombs, that is exactly what you can do! Just draw a bath, add a bomb, and climb in.

Ingredients:

- 1 cup baking soda
- ½ cup Epsom salt
- ½ cup citric acid
- ½ tablespoon olive oil
- ½ tablespoon water
- 1 teaspoon vanilla extract
- ¼ teaspoon each of the following: dried lavender, comfrey, calendula, yarrow flavor, and plantain leaf

Instructions:

1. Stir together the baking soda, Epsom salt, and citric acid in a mixing bowl.
2. In a separate bowl, whisk together the olive oil, water, and vanilla extract.
3. Stir the liquid ingredients into the dry ingredients and mix well by hand until thoroughly combined then stir in the herbs.
4. Add more water, if needed, to make the mixture stick together.

5. Divide the mixture among small silicone molds, pressing it firmly.
6. Let the mold sit for 24 to 48 hours until completely hardened.
7. Remove the bath bombs from the mold and store in an airtight container for up to 2 weeks.
8. To use, add one bath bomb to a hot bath and let it fizz!

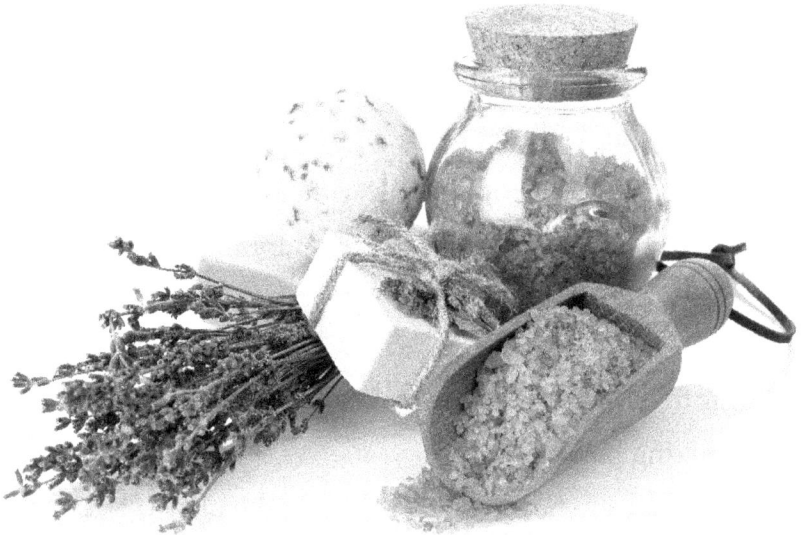

Inflammation-Busting Salt Soak

If you are suffering from sore muscles, bruises, or sprains then this inflammation-busting salt soak may be just what you've been looking for. Draw a hot bath then add some Epsom salt and essential oil then soak the pain away.

Ingredients:

- Hot water, as needed
- 2 cups Epsom salt
- 5 drops lavender essential oil
- 5 drops eucalyptus essential oil

Instructions:

1. Draw a hot bath and, while the water is running, pour in the Epsom salt.
2. Add the essential oils a few drops at a time.
3. Swirl the water gently with your hand to spread the oils and to dissolve the salts.
4. Once the salt is completely dissolved you can turn off the water.
5. Climb into the tub and soak for at least 30 minutes.
6. After soaking for 30 minutes, towel yourself dry. Repeat daily, if needed.

Sunburn-Relieving Spray

After a long day in the sun your skin might feel a little tortured –
especially if you have sunburn. Fortunately, it is easy to tame the
itching and pain that comes with sunburn by using this simple
sunburn-relieving spray. Keep a bottle handy all summer long!

Ingredients:

- 2 tablespoons Epsom salt
- 1 cup warm water
- Empty plastic spray bottle

Instructions:

1. Spoon the Epsom salt into an empty plastic spray bottle.
2. Add the water and shake well to combine.
3. Spritz the mixture over the sunburned area and let it soak in.
4. Repeat the application several times a day, as needed.

Epsom Salt Bath for Tension Headaches

If you are feeling stressed and overworked, it could lead to a tension headache. This Epsom salt bath is the perfect way to relax and unwind while also relieving your headache. Just soak for 30 minutes with your eyes closed and you'll feel brand new!

Ingredients:

- Hot water, as needed
- 2 cups Epsom salt
- 5 drops rosemary essential oil
- 5 drops Roman chamomile essential oil

Instructions:

1. Draw a hot bath and, while the water is running, pour in the Epsom salt.
2. Add the essential oils a few drops at a time.
3. Swirl the water gently with your hand to spread the oils and to dissolve the salts.
4. Once the salt is completely dissolved you can turn off the water.
5. Climb into the tub and soak for at least 30 minutes.
6. After soaking for 30 minutes, towel yourself dry.

Chapped Lip Reliever

Are your lips dry and chapped? If you feel like regular lip balm doesn't work to keep your lips moisturized, try this chapped lip reliever. You won't be disappointed.

Ingredients:

- 2 tablespoons Epsom salt
- 1 teaspoon petroleum jelly
- 3 drops peppermint essential oil

Instructions:

1. Combine the Epsom salt and petroleum jelly in a small bowl.
2. Stir in the peppermint essential oil until well combined.
3. Apply the solution to your lips, gently rubbing it in.
4. Reapply the mixture as needed to relieve pain and dryness.

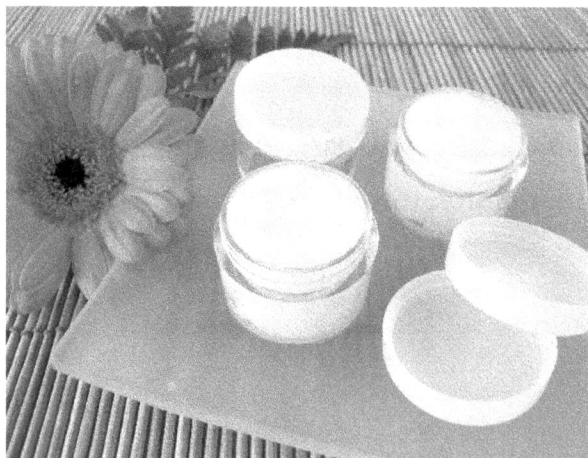

Epsom Salt Soak for Bug Bites

During the summer months it may seem like you are constantly battling bug bites. Fortunately, there is a simple solution for itching and pain relief caused by those bites – just combine some Epsom salt with water and lavender essential oil. It's that easy!

Ingredients:

- 1 cup warm water
- 2 tablespoons Epsom salt
- 2 to 3 drops lavender essential oil

Instructions:

1. Combine the water and Epsom salt in a bowl.
2. Add the essential oil and stir until the salt is dissolved.
3. Dip cotton balls in the mixture than dap them onto the affected area.
4. Let the liquid air-dry and avoid scratching.

Detoxifying Bath Bombs

Over time, toxins and other harmful materials accumulate in your body and they can slow things down. Taking a hot bath with one of these detoxifying bath bombs may help to drain some of those toxins from your body, helping you feel renewed.

Ingredients:

- 1 cup baking soda
- ½ cup Epsom salt
- ½ cup citric acid
- 2 tablespoons coconut oil
- ½ tablespoon water
- 1 teaspoon vanilla extract
- 5 drops lemon essential oil

Instructions:

1. Stir together the baking soda, Epsom salt, and citric acid in a mixing bowl.
2. In a separate bowl, whisk together the coconut oil, water, and vanilla extract.
3. Stir the liquid ingredients into the dry ingredients and mix well by hand until thoroughly combined then stir in the lemon essential oil.
4. Add more water, if needed, to make the mixture stick together.

5. Divide the mixture among small silicone molds, pressing it firmly.
6. Let the mold sit for 24 to 48 hours until completely hardened.
7. Remove the bath bombs from the mold and store in an airtight container for up to 2 weeks.
8. To use, add one bath bomb to a hot bath and let it fizz!

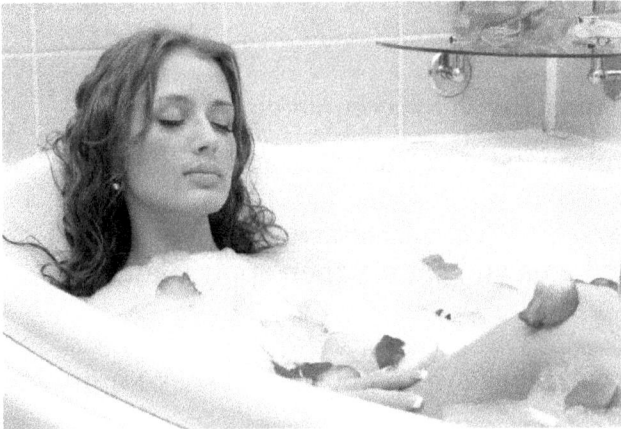

Sore Muscle Soother

Whether you are sore from working out or you just slept in a funny way, this sore muscle soother is the best form of relief you will find – plus, it is all natural!

Ingredients:

- 8 ounces hot water
- 1 teaspoon Epsom salt
- 5 drops sweet marjoram essential oil

Instructions:

1. Pour the water into a small bowl and stir in the Epsom salt and essential oil.
2. Stir the mixture until the salt is completely dissolved.
3. Transfer the solution to the refrigerator and chill for 20 minutes.
4. Clean the affected area and pat dry then apply a layer of paste.
5. Cover the paste with gauze wrapping and let soak for 30 minutes.

Bee Sting Compress

Even if you aren't allergic to bees, bee stings can still be very unpleasant. The last thing you want to do is apply some chemical-based solution to a sensitive area so give this all-natural remedy a try to reduce the swelling and relieve some of the pain.

Ingredients:

- 1 cup cold water
- 2 tablespoons Epsom salt
- 1 drop German chamomile essential oil
- 1 drop peppermint essential oil
- 1 drop lavender essential oil

Instructions:

1. Combine the cold water and Epsom salt in a small bowl.
2. Stir until the salt is dissolved then stir in the essential oil.
3. Soak a washcloth in the solution then lay it over the affected area.
4. Let the washcloth sit on the area until it is no longer cold.
5. Repeat this treatment as needed.

Post-Workout Ice Plunge

After an intense workout your muscles probably feel sore and tired. This post-workout ice plunge is a great way to relieve those feelings while also speeding the recovery process. It may not be pleasant to soak in a tub of ice water but you'll feel great afterward!

Ingredients:

- Cold water, as needed
- Ice cubes, as needed
- ½ cup Epsom salt

Instructions:

1. Fill a bathtub halfway with cold water then add as much ice as you can.
2. Stir in the Epsom salt by hand to distribute it as evenly as possible.
3. Carefully lower yourself into the tub and soak for 20 minutes.

Sleepy Time Epsom Salt Soak

If you have trouble sleeping it may be helpful for you to soak in a hot bath for 30 minutes before bed time. The Epsom salt will help to soothe your body and the aroma from the essential oils will add some extra relaxation power.

Ingredients:

- Hot water, as needed
- 2 cups Epsom salt
- 5 drops Roman chamomile essential oil
- 5 drops lavender essential oil

Instructions:

1. Draw a hot bath and, while the water is running, pour in the Epsom salt.
2. Add the essential oils a few drops at a time.
3. Swirl the water gently with your hand to spread the oils and to dissolve the salts.
4. Once the salt is completely dissolved you can turn off the water.
5. Climb into the tub and soak for at least 30 minutes.
6. After soaking for 30 minutes, towel yourself dry.

Odor and Fungus-Busting Foot Soak

Whether your foot odor is caused by athlete's foot or something else, this odor and fungus-busting foot soak is just what you've been looking for. Just sit back, relax, and let your feet soak for 20 minutes and they'll come out smelling fresh!

Ingredients:

- 2 quarts warm water
- ½ cup Epsom salt
- 4 drops eucalyptus essential oil
- 4 drops sweet orange essential oil

Instructions:

1. Pour two quarts of warm water into a basin then stir in the Epsom salt.
2. Add the essential oils and swirl well to distribute.
3. Place the basin on the floor and soak your feet for 15 to 20 minutes.
4. Remove your feet from the basin and scrub your feet well with an Epsom salt scrub.
5. Rinse your feet well with warm water then towel dry.

Home and Garden Epsom Salt Recipes

Toilet-Cleaning Bombs

If you hate cleaning the toilet, these toilet-cleaning bombs will become your best friend. Just drop one into the toilet and give it a quick scrub then flush!

Ingredients:

- 1 cup baking soda
- 1/3 cup citric acid
- 2 tablespoons Epsom salt
- 30 drops lemon essential oil
- 20 drops orange essential oil

Instructions:

1. Stir together the baking soda, Epsom salt, and citric acid in a mixing bowl.
2. Spritz the mixture with water to dampen and mix well by hand until thoroughly combined.
3. Add more water, if needed, to make the mixture stick together.
4. Stir in the essential oils and keep mixing until it just comes together.
5. Spoon the mixture onto a parchment-lined baking sheet in rounded tablespoons.

6. Let the tray sit for 24 to 48 hours until completely hardened.
7. Remove the bombs from the mold and store in an airtight container for up to 2 weeks.
8. T use, simply drop one of these bombs into the bowl and let it fizz then scrub clean.

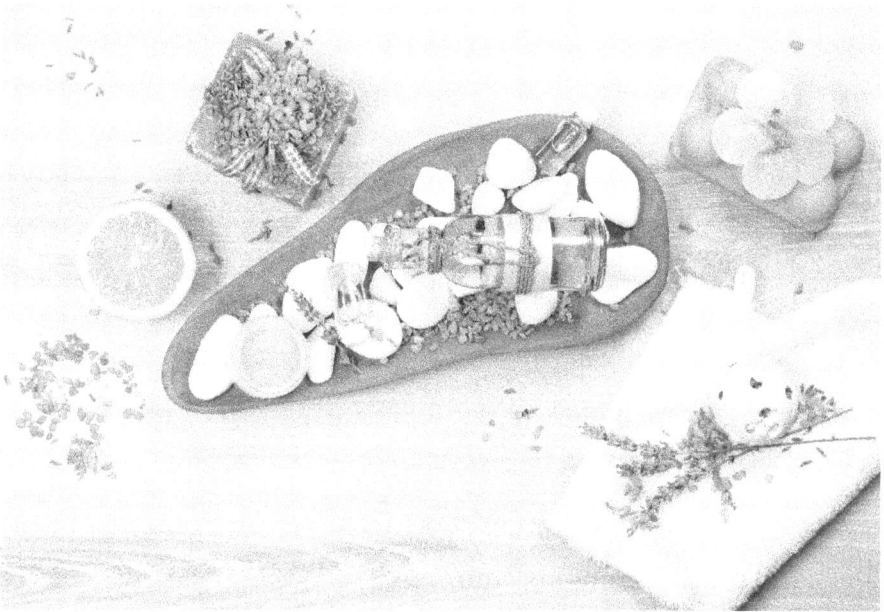

Grime-Busting Salt Scrub

Do you have dishes or baking equipment that is marred by baked-on food or stubborn stains? Rather than throwing these things out, just use Epsom salt to scrub them! You will be amazed at how simple and effective this remedy can be.

Ingredients:

- Warm water, as needed
- 1 teaspoon Epsom salt

Instructions:

1. Fill a sink with warm water.
2. Add about 1 teaspoon of Epsom salt and stir until it dissolves.
3. Place your dishes in the sink and let them soak for 5 minutes.
4. Take a scrub brush or an abrasive sponge and scrub the baked-on food away.
5. Rinse the dishes then let them air dry.

Simple Tile Scrubber

Kitchen and bathroom tiles can get very dirty very quickly and, unfortunately, they are often very hard to clean. With this simple tile scrubber, however, you will find that your kitchen and bathroom cleanup is quicker and easier than ever!

Ingredients:

- ¼ cup mild dish soap
- ¼ cup Epsom salt
- 10 drops lemon essential oil
- 5 drops lime essential oil

Instructions:

1. Combine the dish soap and Epsom salt in a small bowl.
2. Add the essential oil then stir until thoroughly combined.
3. Apply the mixture to your tiles by hand or with a brush.
4. Scrub the mixture into the tile until it is clean then rinse well.

Green Garden Epsom Salt Remedy

Do you want your lawn to be lush and green but you don't want to use expensive chemical fertilizers? You will be glad to know that Epsom salt is a highly effective fertilizer! You can use it on grass or any other plants for a boost of nutrition.

Ingredients:

- Epsom salt, as needed
- Water, as needed

Instructions:

1. Sprinkle the Epsom salt over your lawn or at the base of your plants.
2. Water the plants to help the Epsom salt soak into the soil.
3. Repeat this treatment once a month for the best results.

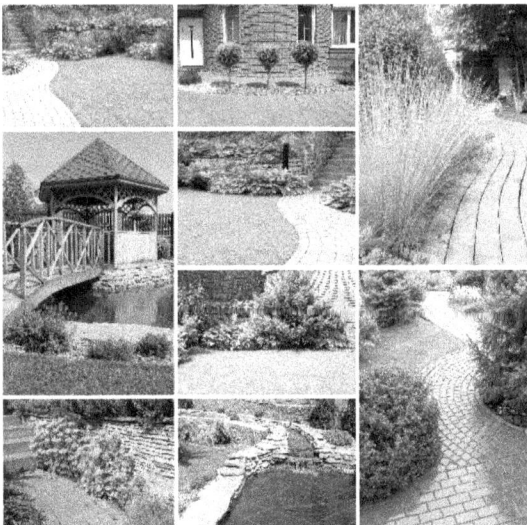

Raccoon Repellant

If you live in an area where raccoons are a problem you may feel as though you have tried everything to keep these pesky critters out of your garbage. What you may not realize is that the simple solution has been in front of you all along – Epsom salt!

Ingredients:

- Epsom salt, as needed

Instructions:

1. Make sure your trash containers have lids on them.
2. Sprinkle a circle of Epsom salt around your trash containers – raccoons do not like the smell so they will avoid the area.

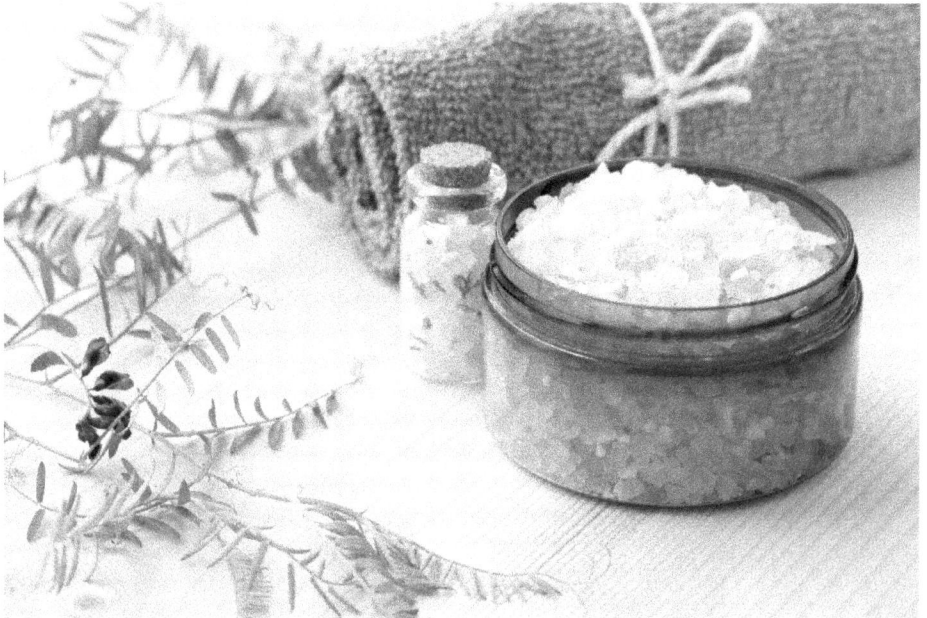

Big Blooming Rose Treatment

If you have a green thumb you may find that you want to try your hand at growing roses. Rose bushes can be a little finicky sometimes but using Epsom salt when you plant your bushes for the first time can help them grow big and beautiful.

Ingredients:

- Epsom salt, as needed

Instructions:

1. Dig the hole where you want to plant your rose bush.
2. Sprinkle a little bit of Epsom salt into the hole.
3. Place the plant in the hole and backfill it with dirt.
4. Pack the soil in around the roots and water the plant well.

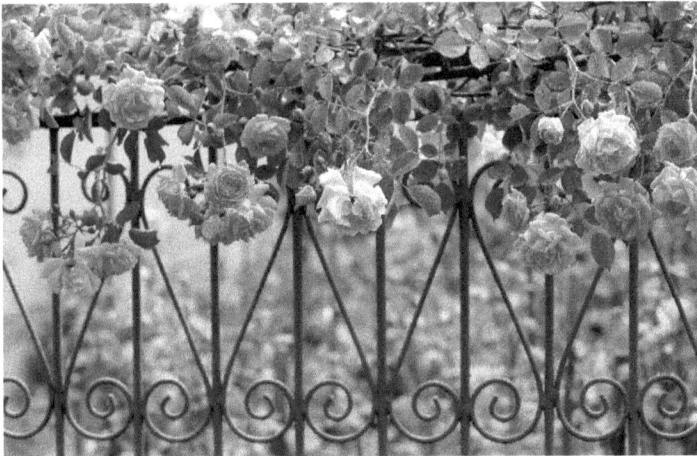

Skin-Softening Hand Wash

If you are tired of harsh liquid soaps that dry out your hands you will be glad to know that there is a better solution. This skin-softening hand wash is made with Epsom salt, baby oil, and essential oils so it works great and smells wonderful.

Ingredients:

- 2 tablespoons Epsom salt
- 1 cup baby oil
- 3 drops jasmine essential oil
- 3 drops vanilla essential oil

Instructions:

1. Combine the Epsom salt and baby oil in a mixing bowl.
2. Stir the mixture until well combined.
3. Pour the soap into an empty plastic bottle and keep by the sink.
4. Use the soap to wash your hands as needed.

Washing Machine Refresher

Your washing machine is supposed to help you keep your clothes clean, but over time the machine itself can become dirty. The more laundry you do, the more detergent buildup you will find inside your washer. This simple washing machine refresher will help get rid of it.

Ingredients:

- ½ cup Epsom salt

Instructions:

1. Fill your washing machine tub with hot water.
2. Add the Epsom salt and give it a moment to dissolve.
3. Set the washing machine to agitate or soak and let it run.
4. Let the washing machine run its course then check to see the results.

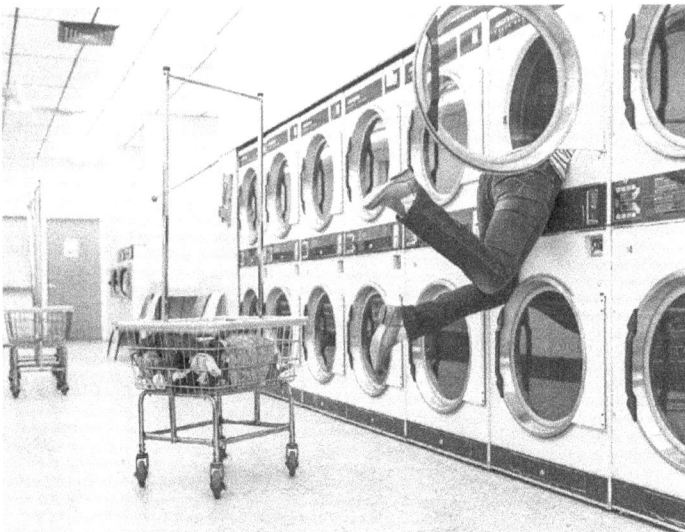

Natural Insecticide Spray

Do you struggle with insect pests feeding on your favorite garden plants? This all-natural insecticide spray is a simple but effective alternative to chemical pesticides. Just mix up a batch and spritz it into your plants for maximum protection.

Ingredients:

- 2 tablespoons Epsom salt
- 16 ounces warm water
- 5 drops lemon essential oil
- 5 drops citronella essential oil
- 5 drops tea tree essential oil

Instructions:

1. Pour the Epsom salts into a large plastic spray bottle.
2. Fill the bottle with warm water then shake until the salts dissolve.
3. Add the essential oils then shake well to combine.
4. Spritz the mixture liberally over your plants to protect them against insect pests.

Deodorizing Kitchen Sink Rinse

Even if you clean your kitchen sink regularly, odors can still buildup in the plumbing – especially if you have a garbage disposal. Fortunately, tackling those tough odors is as simple as mixing some Epsom salt with a little hot water and some essential oils.

Ingredients:

- 4 cups hot water
- 1 cup Epsom salt
- 10 drops lemon essential oil
- 10 drops eucalyptus essential oil

Instructions:

1. Combine the hot water and Epsom salt in a mixing bowl.
2. Stir until the salts dissolve then stir in the essential oils.
3. Clean your kitchen sink to remove residue then pour the mixture down the drain.
4. Run the hot water in the sink to help flush out the odor.

Easy Refrigerator Cleaner

When it comes to cleaning your refrigerator, deodorizing is just as important as sanitizing. This recipe for easy refrigerator cleaner harnesses the cleaning power of Epsom salt with the deodorizing power of lemon juice and baking soda.

Ingredients:

- 3 cups warm water
- 1 cup distilled white vinegar
- 2 tablespoons baking soda
- 2 tablespoons Epsom salt
- 20 drops lemon essential oil

Instructions:

1. Pour the water into a bowl.
2. Add the vinegar, baking soda, Epsom salt, and essential oils.
3. Stir everything together until the salt is completely dissolved.
4. Transfer the mixture to an empty plastic spray bottle.
5. Spritz the mixture into your refrigerator and wipe clean with a damp sponge.

Coffee Pot Cleaner

The more you use your coffee pot, the dirtier it gets. Even if you wash it every day, however, it never seems to be completely clean. If you want your coffee pot to look and smell like new, give this simple coffee pot cleaner a try.

Ingredients:

- 2 tablespoons Epsom salt
- Ice cubes, as needed
- 1 lemon, cut into wedges

Instructions:

1. Sprinkle the Epsom salt into the coffee pot.
2. Add a handful of ice cubes and some lemon wedges.
3. Swirl the ingredient around inside the coffee pot for a few minutes.
4. Dump out the ingredients then rinse the pot clean.

Cutting Board Scrubber

To keep your cutting board in good condition you should always wash it by hand. Unfortunately, it can be difficult to get a deep clean if your cutting board is covered with scratches. This cutting board scrubber is a quick and easy way to clean your cutting board without putting it through the dishwasher.

Ingredients:

- Epsom salt, as needed
- 1 lemon, cut in half

Instructions:

1. Rinse the cutting board to remove food residue.
2. While the cutting board is still damp, sprinkle it with Epsom salt.
3. Cut the lemon in half and use one half to scrub the cutting board – the Epsom salt will help to scrub away residue while the lemon kills germs.
4. Use the second half of the lemon, if needed, then rinse and let air-dry.

Artificial Flower Arranger

If you like to make your own artificial flower arrangements at home you might already have a preference for what you use to keep the flowers in place. If you want to ditch the green foam and use something that looks nice, try using some Epsom salt and water.

Ingredients:

- Epsom salt, as needed
- Water, as needed
- Artificial flowers

Instructions:

1. Pour the Epsom salt into the vase or whatever container you are using for your arrangement.
2. Add enough water to dampen the salt then arrange your flowers as desired.
3. As the salt dries, it will harden which will hold the flowers in place.

Conclusion

By now it should be clear to you that Epsom salts are an amazing thing. While they may not technically be a salt, there are an unlimited array of options for how to use this wonderful material. Whether you are looking for a way to relax and unwind after a long day or want to create your own homemade cleaning products, Epsom salts are the way to go! In reading this book you have received an in-depth overview of what Epsom salts are and how they can be used, so you are probably eager to try some of these solutions for yourself. If you are, don't delay any longer – pick a recipe and give it a try for yourself!

As a last note, it is once again very necessary to <u>remind you that all of the products and recipes in this book should be used with absolute caution and that if any irritation or sensitivity is experienced due to the use of any of these products it is very strongly advised that you discontinue use of the product immediately</u>. Furthermore if any reaction to any of the products or recipes in this book does not clear up within three days of the discontinuation of use of the product, it is strongly advised that you consult with your doctor or dermatologist.

Finally, if you have a second, please review this book on Amazon.

Even one sentence review will do and I'd be really happy to hear from you!

I hope you will enjoy your holistic health and beauty journey!

I hope to "see" you in my next book.

You may also be interested in Cassia's book:

"Homemade Beauty Products: Easy DIY Recipes & Holistic Solutions for Glowing Skin and Beautiful Hair".

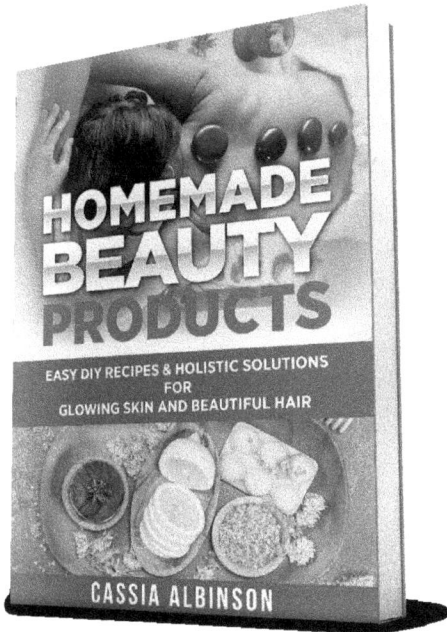

You will find it in your local Amazon Store (Kindle and Paperback)

Visit:

www.HolisticWellnessBooks.com

for more!

AROMATHERAPY & ESSENTIAL OILS PRECAUTIONS

Aromatherapy General Precautions

Aromatherapy is a very safe and easy therapy to use, but keep in mind that there are certain precautions:

- Remember to wash your hands after applying aromatherapy massage;

- Do not apply the essential oils in their pure form as they may cause an allergic reaction. Instead, use blends that contain 2-5% essential oils diluted in good-quality cold-pressed oil;

-After using citrus oils, like for example lemon, verbena, bergamot, orange etc. avoid direct sun exposure, even up to 8 hours after the treatment

- Do not apply oils after surgery (unless you have consulted with a doctor) or on open wounds or rashes of unknown origin;

- Do not use the oils after chemotherapy (unless suggested by a doctor);

- Keep the oils away from the eyes and mucus membranes;

- Use the oils only topically (unless you have consulted with an aromatherapist who specializes in phytoaromatherapy);

- Avoid rosemary, thyme, Spanish and common sage, fennel and hyssop if you suffer from high blood pressure;

- Do not apply the treatments described in this book on babies or infants. It doesn't mean that aromatherapy can never be used on babies and infants, but extremely low concentrations should be used. Always consult with a medical or naturopathy doctor first;

- After an aromatherapy massage always remember to wash your hands;

- Make sure that you research the brand, read safety instructions for each individual oil you buy/use and check the expiration date;

- Store your blends in dark glass bottles, preferably in a cool, dry and dark place and remember to use within a maximum of one month after mixing.

www.ingramcontent.com/pod-product-compliance
Lightning Source LLC
Chambersburg PA
CBHW051037030426
42336CB00015B/2926